Math for Healthcare Professions

2ND EDITION

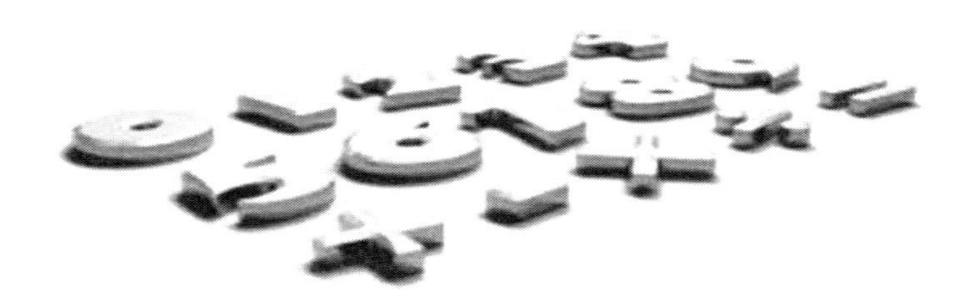

Louie Asuncion

USN Ret, BS (Health Care Management),
MBA (Healthcare Administration),
Associate Professor, Health Occupations

Del Mar College

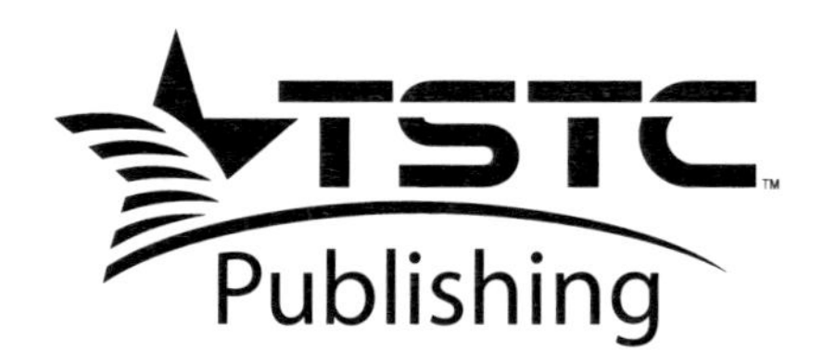

ISBN 978-1-936603-09-1 (softback)
ISBN 978-1-934302-80-4 (ebook)

TSTC Publishing
Texas State Technical College Waco
3801 Campus Drive
Waco, TX 76705

http://publishing.tstc.edu/

Publisher: Mark Long
Editor: Ana Wraight
Art director: Stacie Buterbaugh
Marketing: Sheila Boggess
Sales: Wes Lowe
Office coordinator: Melanie Peterson
Cover design: Brooke Hernandez
Book design & layout: Adam Chumley
Printing production: Bill Evridge

Manufactured in the United States of America

Second edition

This book is dedicated to my loving family

Table of Contents

Chapter One: Roman Numerals

Roman numerals are used to express numerical value in the apothecary system of measurement. Note that it is rare to use numbers higher than 45 in the apothecary system; however, principles in writing and reading Roman numerals remain the same.

All numbers are written in terms of addition and subtraction of letters. Common letters used in the Roman numeral system and their equivalent in the Arabic number system are:

ss = ½
I or i = 1
V = 5
X = 10
L = 50
C = 100
D = 500
M = 1000

Principles

1) If a small value letter is written after the same letter or a larger value letter, the value of the smaller letter is added to the value of the preceding larger letter. However, when you add, you can only add up to 3 of the same consecutive letter.

   XIII = 10+1+1+1 = 13

2) If a small value letter is written before a larger value letter, the value of the smaller letter is subtracted to the value of the larger letter. However, when you subtract, you can only subtract the value of 1 small letter from the value of the larger letter.

   IV = 5-1 = 4

3) In properly writing a Roman numeral, each column (1s, 10s, 100s, 1000s ...) has to be represented by the specific Roman numeral for that column.

   1 9 9
   C XC IX

***Note:** In deciphering Roman numerals, use the same principles but in the opposite manner (start from the right to left direction).

Exercises

Express in Roman numerals:

1. 14 ____________
2. 8 1/2 ____________
3. 36 _______________
4. 25 _______________

Express in Arabic numbers:

5. XIII ___________
6. XXIXss ___________
7. XLII ___________
8. XXXVIII ___________

Chapter Two: Fractions

A fraction represents a part of a whole (number). It is commonly used in healthcare. It has a numerator and a denominator.

$$\frac{3 \text{ (numerator)}}{4 \text{ (denominator)}}$$

The line between the numerator and the denominator may mean divide or ratio. The numerator tells us how many parts we are talking about, and the denominator tells how many equal parts a whole is subdivided into.

Common Types of Fractions

Proper

A fraction in which the numerator is smaller than the denominator (1/3)

Improper

A fraction in which the numerator is larger than the denominator (5/3)

Whole Number

A fraction that has an unexpressed denominator of one (2/1, 3/1)

Mixed Number

A whole number and a fraction together (2 ½, 3 ½)

Complex Fraction

A fraction in which the numerator has a fraction, the denominator have a fraction, or the numerator and denominator has fractions:

$$\frac{\frac{1}{2}}{2}, \frac{3}{\frac{1}{2}}, \frac{\frac{1}{2}}{\frac{1}{3}}$$

Comparing Size of Fractions (Larger or Smaller)

Principles

1) If the numerators are "1" or the same, the fraction whose denominator is smaller is the larger:

1/6 is larger than 1/9

2) If the denominators are the same, the fraction whose numerator is larger is the larger:

3/5 is larger than 1/5

If the numerators are not the same and the denominators are not the same, find the common denominator first, preferably the least common denominator (LCD). To find the LCD of fractions, find the smallest number that can be divided by both denominators of the terms evenly (without remainder).

The LCD of the fractions 3/6 and 4/12 is 6.

Transition of the Common Types of Fractions

An improper fraction can be changed to a whole or mixed number by dividing the numerator by the denominator.

$8/3 = 8 \div 3 = 2\ 2/3$

A mixed number can be changed to an improper fraction by multiplying the denominator of the fraction to the whole number, adding the numerator, and then retaining the denominator of the fraction.

$$1\ 3/4 = \frac{(4 \times 1) + 3}{4} = \frac{7}{4}$$

To reduce a fraction to its lowest term, find the largest number that can divide |both the numerator and denominator of the term evenly (in this example, the number is 6).

$$\frac{6}{12} = \frac{6 \div 6}{12 \div 6} = \frac{1}{2}$$

To find the LCD without changing the value of the fraction, find the smallest number that can be divided by the denominator of each term evenly (in this case it is 10), then multiply the quotient by the numerator of each term. Retain the common denominator.

1/5 The LCD of these terms is 10.

and

1/10 Therefore, 1/5 = 2/10 and 1/10 remains the same.

Operation of Fractions

In the operation of fractions, the following steps are strongly recommended:

1) Analyze the terms to see if any can be reduced to their lowest term
2) Reduce to the lowest term (simplify)
3) Change mixed numbers to improper fractions
4) Find the common denominator (preferably the LCD)
5) Proceed with the required operation

Addition and Subtraction

Principle

Before adding or subtracting fractions, they must be of the same denominators (preferably the LCD). Add or subtract numerators and retain the common denominator.

2 ½ + 1 4/12 - 3/12 = ?

2 ½ + 1 1/3 (simplified) - ¼ (simplified) =

5/2 (changed into improper fraction) + 4/3 (changed into improper fraction) – ¼ =

5/2 + 4/3 - ¼ = ?   * The LCD is 12.

$$\frac{30}{12} + \frac{16}{12} - \frac{3}{12} = \frac{43}{12} \text{ or } 3\ 7/12$$

Multiplication

Principle

In the multiplication of fractions, follow steps 1 – 3 and 5 above. Multiply numerators together, multiply denominators together, and then reduce to the lowest term as appropriate.

2 ½ X 1 8/24 =

$$\frac{5}{2} \text{ X } 1\ 1/3 = \frac{5}{2} \text{ X } \frac{4}{3} = \frac{20}{6} \text{ simplified to } \frac{10}{3} \text{ or } 3\ 1/3$$

Division

Principle

In the division of fractions, follow the previous steps 1 – 3 and 5. Take the first term (or numerator), take the inverse or reciprocal of the second term (or denominator), change the division sign to a multiplication sign, and proceed as multiplication.

$$\frac{2\frac{1}{2}}{2} = \frac{\frac{5}{2}}{2} = \frac{5}{2} \text{ X } \frac{1}{2} \text{ (the reciprocal of } \frac{2}{1} \text{)} = \frac{5}{4}$$

Transition of Fractions

Fractions are expressions of ratios, decimals, and percentages.

1) To express a fraction as a ratio, write the numerator, place a colon (:) after, then write the denominator:

   1/4 = 1 :4 in ratio form

2) To express a fraction as a decimal, divide the numerator by the denominator:

   1/4 = (1 divided by 4) = 0 .25

3) To express a decimal as a percent, move the decimal place 2 places to the right and add a percent (%) sign:

   .5 = 50 % , .25 = 25 %

4) To express a percent as a decimal, move the decimal place 2 places to the left and remove the percent sign:

   50. % = .5 , 25.% = .25

5) To express a percent as a fraction, simply remove the percent sign and write this number as the numerator. Then, use 100 as the denominator, reduce as needed:

   $50\,\% = \frac{50}{100} = \frac{1}{2}$, $25\,\% = \frac{25}{100} = \frac{1}{4}$

6) To express a decimal as a fraction, properly read the decimal as you write the equivalent fraction. (Remember the columns in decimal numbers, i.e. tenths, hundredths, thousandths, etc.)

.1 is read and written as one tenth (1/10)
.12 is read and written as twelve hundredths (12/100)
.123 is read and written as one hundred twenty three thousandths

(123/1000)

Exercises

Reduce the following fractions to the lowest terms:

1. 15/25 ___________ 3. 12/52 ___________

2. 8/28 ___________ 4. 20/55 ___________

Change the following improper fractions to whole or mixed numbers. Reduce to the lowest terms:

5. 11/2 ___________ 7. 17/7 ___________

6. 17/6 ___________ 8. 13/8 ___________

Change the following mixed numbers to improper fractions:

9. 3 5/9 ___________ 11. 5 3/16 ___________

10. 6 4/13 ___________ 12. 8 5/14 ___________

Circle the larger fraction in each pair:

13. 6/13 or 9/13

14. 3/7 or 8/11

15. 8/11 or 8/19

16. 4/15 or 6/7

Circle the smaller fraction in each pair:

17. 8/17 or 4/17

18. 2/11 or 2/13

19. 6/13 or 7/16

Add the following fractions and mixed numbers, and reduce to the lowest terms:

20. 4 2/5
 2 1/2
 + 3/4

21. 4 2/3
 1/4
 + 5/6

22. 9 2/3
 3 2/5
 + 3/4

Subtract the following fractions:

23. 2 1/4
 - 1 1/3

24. 5 1/2
 - 1 1/3

25. 6 1/4
 - 6 1/6

Multiply the following fractions and mixed numbers:

26. 3 5/6 x 4 1/8 = ___________

27. 2 1/6 x 5 ½ = ___________

28. 1 2/4 x 7 = ___________

29. 5 1/3 x 2 6/8 = ___________

Fraction word problems:

30. A clinic purchased an electronic vital signs equipment for $2,000 with a yearly maintenance cost of 1/5 of the purchase price. How much is the annual maintenance cost for this equipment?

31. A patient weighs 150 pounds (lb). If he is to receive 5 milligrams (mg) of medication per 50 pounds of body weight, how many mg of medication will be prescribed?

Chapter Three: Decimals and Percents

Decimals are expressions of fractions, ratios, and percentages.

Addition

Principle

In the addition of decimals, the decimal place in the sum or total (result of addition) must be in the same column as in the addends (numbers being added):

```
       .13
(+)    .012
      -----
       .142
```

Subtraction

Principle

In the subtraction of decimals, the decimal place in the remainder or difference (result of subtraction) must be in the same column as in the subtrahends (numbers being subtracted):

```
       .13
(-)    .012
      -----
       .118
```

Multiplication

Principle

In multiplying decimals, the number of decimal places in the product (result of multiplication) must be equal to the number of decimal places in the multiplicand and multiplier (numbers being multiplied):

```
       .13
(x)    .012
      ------
       .00156
```

Division

Principle

In dividing decimals, first convert the divisor (number dividing with) into a whole number (move decimal place to the right, after the number), then move the same number of decimal places in the dividend (number being divided).

Proceed as if dividing whole numbers with the decimal place in the quotient (result of division) on the same column as in the dividend:

.015 $\div$ .15 can be expressed as $\frac{1.5}{15} = 0.1$

Percentage Problem

Mixtures and solutions are common in healthcare. Therefore, a basic knowledge of percentage (strength) problems is important as it affects patient treatment outcome. ("Of" means to multiply):

.15% of 20 = ?

15% of 40 = ?

The first step is to convert the percentage to its decimal form by moving the decimal place 2 places to the left. Then and only then should you proceed with multiplication:

$.0015 \times 20 = 0.03$

***Note:** The movements of 2 decimal places to the left and removal of the % sign before multiplying.

$.15 \times 40 = 6$

Or, write the percent as a fraction (remove the percent sign and use 100 as the denominator). Proceed as in multiplication/division of fractions/decimals.

$$\frac{.15}{100} \times 20 = \frac{.15}{5} = 0.03$$

$$\frac{15}{100} \times 40 = \frac{(15)(2)}{5} = 6$$

Exercises

Change the following decimals to fractions, and reduce to the lowest terms:

1. 0.125 = ____________
2. 0.45 = ____________
3. 0.635 = ____________
4. 0.007 = ____________

Circle the larger of the two decimals:

5. 0.3 or 0.06

6. 0.02 or 0.025

7. .12 or 0.078

Rewrite the following fractions as ratios, percentages, and decimals:

FRACTION	RATIO	PERCENTAGE	DECIMAL
8. 2/5	= __________	= __________	= __________
9. 2/9	= __________	= __________	= __________
10. 8/28	= __________	= __________	= __________
11. 6/15	= __________	= __________	= __________

Solve the following percentage problems:

12. 6% of 85 = __________

13. 0.8% of 132 = __________

14. 1.8% of 28 = __________

15. 0.09% of 68 = __________

Percentage word problems:

16. A Hydrocortisone Cream has 2 milligrams (mg) of hydrocortisone per 100 mg of the compound. What is the actual percentage of hydrocortisone in the compound?

17. An Intravenous solution of D5RL has 5 grams (g) of dextrose in each of 100 mL solution. What is the percentage of Ringer's lactate in the solution?

Chapter Four: Ratios and Proportions

Ratio

The relationship between two quantities or numbers, to a whole (of which one has a bearing on the other) is a ratio. In other words, if one number changes, the other number must also change. The relationship is designated by a colon (:) between the numbers.

1 : 3

***Note:** Remember that a ratio can also be expressed as a fraction $\left(\frac{1}{3}\right)$

Proportion

The relationship between two (2) equal ratios is a proportion. The relationship may be designated by two sets of colon (: :) between the numbers or as equal ratios.

1 : 3 : : 4 : 2 OR $\frac{1}{3} = \frac{4}{2}$

Application

Principle

The product of the means is equal to the product of the extremes (or the cross-products are equal). The means are the second and the third numbers in a proportion relationship. The extremes are the first and fourth numbers in a proportion relationship.

Means Extremes

(3) x (4) = (1) x (2)

Ratio and proportion may be used in solving problems of one unknown, as in unit conversions by solving for the unknown X.

Problem: 1:3 :: 4:X

Product of the means (3) (4) = Product of the extremes (1) (X)

Therefore, (3) (4) = (1) (X) , hence, X = 12

Problem: 3 : 2 :: X : 1.5

$$(2)(X) = (3)(1.5)$$
$$2X = 4.5$$
$$\frac{2X}{2} = \frac{4.5}{2}$$

***Note:** Division of both sides by the coefficient of X, which is 2

Therefore, $X = 2.25$

Problem: $\frac{1}{150} : \frac{1}{200} :: 1 : X$

$$(1/150)(X) = (1)(1/200)$$

$$\frac{X}{150} = \frac{1}{200}$$

$$(150)\frac{X}{150} = \frac{1}{200}(150)$$ (Multiply both sides by the reciprocal of the coefficient of X, which is 150)

Therefore, $X = \frac{150}{200} = \frac{3}{4}$

Solving Unit Conversion Problems with Ratio and Proportion

Problem: 1 L = ________________ mL

The problem itself is the first ratio, X being the unknown: (1 : X)

The second ratio is from the conversion chart: 1L = 1000 mL (1 : 1000)

Therefore, $1 : X :: 1 : 1000$

$$(X)(1) = (1)(1000)$$

$$X = 1000 \text{ mL}$$

Problem: 5 Kg = ___lbs 1 Kg = 2.2 lbs

$$5 : X :: 1 : 2.2$$

$$(X)(1) = (5)(2.2)$$

$$X = 11.0 \text{ lbs}$$

Problem: 2 pt = ___ oz 1 pt = 16 oz

$$2 : X :: 1 : 16$$

$$(X)(1) = (2)(16)$$

$$X = 32 \text{ oz}$$

Problem: 1000 mL = ___oz where 30 mL = 1 oz

$$1000 : X :: 30 : 1$$

$$(X)(30) = (1000)(1)$$

$$30X = 1000$$

$$X = \frac{1000}{30}$$

$$X = 33.33 \text{ oz}$$

Problem: .003 Kg = ___mg 1 Kg = 1000 g

.003 : X :: 1 : 1000
(X) (1) = (.003) (1000)
X = 3 g (Not in milligrams yet)

Continuing, 3 g = ___ mg 1 g = 1000 mg

3 : X :: 1 : 1000
(X) (1) = (3) (1000)
X = 3000 mg

Exercises

Solve for "X" in the following proportions:

1. 2 : 7 :: 5 : X/2

2. 1/2 : X :: 2/3 : 12

3. X/15 = 7/20

4. 13X : 3 :: 1/3 : 1/26

5. 3/4 = 5X/1.5

6. 3 : 14 :: 3/4 : X/3

7. X/5 = 3/8

8. 4/22 = 6/ X/2

9. 5 : 13 :: X/2 : 17

10. 8 : 12 :: 5 : 3X

Unit conversion word problems:

11. How many teaspoons (tsp) are in 1 pint of medication preparation?

12. If there are 12 mg in a tablespoon (Tbs) of cough syrup, how many mg are in 5 fluid ounces (oz)?

13. A physician orders a tsp of oral medication twice a day. How many days will ½ of a pint last?

14. If a man weighs 220 pounds (lb), what is his weight in kilograms (kg)?

15. If a patient is to take 10 grains (gr) of aspirin for his headache, how many milligrams (mg) is he to take?

Chapter 5: Dimensional Analysis

Dimensional analysis is a systematic problem-solving method. It is often referred to as the problem-solving method of choice because it provides a straightforward way to set up problems; gives a clear understanding of the principles of the problem; helps the learner to organize, visualize, and evaluate data; assists in determining whether the setup of the problem is correct; and even confirms that you have arrived at the answer to the problem. It is less prone to errors than solving problems by the ratio and proportion methods. It is most often used when two quantities are directly proportional to each other in the system of measurements, as in chemistry. This approach to solving conversion problems works on a fraction method.

There are four elements required to facilitate this problem solving method. Once the (1) given quantity is known, the (2) required quantity identified, the (3) unit paths leading from what is given to what is required is established, and the (4) corresponding conversion factor(s) for each unit path(s) identified; the problem-solving method of dimensional analysis can be readily applied.

The following example illustrates the steps to solve a problem using dimensional analysis.

Example

1 liter (L) equals how many ounces (oz)? How many ounces are in 1 L?
(1 L = _____oz)

Step 1: Identify the given quantity in the problem. (The given quantity is 1 L)

Step 2: Identify what is required. (oz)

Step 3: Establish unit path. (L to mL, then mL to oz)

Step 4: Determine the specific conversion factor for each unit path. (1L = 1000 mL)
(30 mL = 1 oz)

Step 5: Set up the problem in fraction format to facilitate the cancellation of units. Each conversion factor is a ratio of unit that equals 1. The conversion factors are set up to cancel out the preceding unit. The given quantity and wanted quantity must be within the numerator portion of the problem to confirm that the problem is set up correctly. Carefully choose each conversion factor and ensure that it is correctly placed in the numerator or denominator portion of the problem to allow the unwanted units to be canceled from the problem. If you are unable to cancel unwanted units because both units are numerators or denominators, then the problem is not set up correctly. The units need to be on opposite side of the fraction (division) line.

Step 6: Multiply numerators together and multiply denominators together.

Step 7: Proceed with division of the resulting numerator by the denominator to obtain numerical value.

$$\frac{1\text{ L}}{} \quad \frac{1000\text{ mL}}{1\text{ L}} \quad \frac{1\text{ oz}}{30\text{ mL}}$$

***Note:** (L and mL cancel out)

$$\frac{1 \times 1000 \times 1}{30} = \frac{1000}{30} = 33.33\text{ oz}$$

***Note:** (oz is the only remaining unit)

Exercises

1. Problem: ¾ mL = How many m? ___________

2. Problem: gtt XV = How many m? ___________

3. Problem: 5/6 gr = How many mg? ___________

4. Problem: How many mL in 3 oz? ___________

5. Problem: 0.5 mg = How many mcg? ___________

6. Problem: 35 gtt = How many mL? ___________

7. Problem: How many cc in 3 qt? ___________

8. Problem: 4 gal = How many qt? ___________

9. Problem: 1.5 cup = How many cc? ___________

10. Problem: 24 oz = How many glasses? ___________

Convert the following to the equivalent measures indicated:

11. 0.002 kg = ___________ mg
12. 6.5 tbs = ___________ oz
13. 220 lbs = ___________ Kg
14. gr iiiss = ___________ mg
15. 0.480 L = ___________ pt
16. 3½ tbs = ___________ tsp
17. 0.135 L = ___________ mL
18. 60 gtts = ___________ tsp
19. 96°F = ___________ °C
20. 17.5 cm = ___________ in
21. 7 mL = ___________ gtts
22. 150 mg = ___________ g

23. 35.4 °C = ___________ °F
24. 45 mL = ___________ dr
25. dr xxviiss = ___________ m
26. 103.6 °F = ___________ °C
27. 84 lbs = ___________ Kg
28. 120 cm = ___________ in
29. 4 qt = ___________ mL
30. 3.05 g = ___________ mg
31. 0.45 g = ___________ gr
32. 44°C = ___________ °F
33. 65 Kg = ___________ lbs
34. 3.5 qt = ___________ L

Chapter 6: Time Conversions

Nowadays, it is common practice in healthcare to use the twenty-four hour (24-Hr) format in documenting care and events. It is, therefore, imperative that a healthcare worker be adept in converting standard time format to this 24-Hr format and vice versa.

Principle

In converting standard time to 24-Hr time (also called military time), the time before 1:00 PM remains the same but is written in four digits (minutes remain the same). The time starting at 1:00 PM and ending at 12:00 midnight has 1200 added to it.

Example

5:30 AM = 0530

9:10 AM = 0910

***Note:** When a 24-Hr time starts with 0, it is understood to be morning (AM).

1:00 PM = 1300 (100 + 1200)

2:15 PM = 1415 (215 + 1200)

***Note:** All times are written the same until 12:59 PM. When time turns to 1:00 PM, 1200 is added (minutes remain the same).

12:00 AM = 2400 (1200 + 1200)

Principle

When converting a 24-Hr time to standard time, the time before 1300 remains the same; however, it is now required to have the designations AM (ante meridian) or PM (post meridian) as appropriate. The time starting at 1300 to 2400 will have 1200 subtracted from it.

0615 = 6:15 AM
0920 = 9:20 AM
1259 = 12:59 PM

1300 = 1:00 PM (1300 - 1200)
1415 = 2:15 PM (1415 - 1200)
2359 = 11:59 PM (2359 - 1200)

Exercises

Convert from traditional times to 24-Hr time or vice versa:

1. 10:45 pm = ___________ hrs.
2. 12:00 (midnight) = ___________ hrs.
3. 5:27 am = ___________ hrs.
4. 11:15 am = ___________ hrs.
5. 0215 hrs. = ___________
6. 2355 hrs. = ___________
7. 1020 hrs. = ___________
8. 1530 hrs. = ___________

Chapter 7: Temperature Conversions

Reporting of temperatures in healthcare varies from institution to institution. For example, some may require temperatures to be reported in degrees Celsius (°C), and some may require it in degrees Fahrenheit (°F). Therefore, a healthcare worker needs to know how to convert one to the other and vice versa. It is simply substituting the letters in the formula and carrying out, required operation.

Formula for converting from °F to °C :

$$°C = (°F - 32) \times 5/9$$

Formula for converting from °C to °F :

$$°F = [(°C)(9/5)] + 32$$

Example: 100 °C = __________ ° F

$$°F = [(100)(9/5)] + 32 = 180 + 32 = 212\ °F$$

Example: 212 °F = __________ °C

$$°C = (212 - 32) \times 5/9 = (180) \times (5/9) = 100\ °C$$

*Note: In healthcare, temperatures are normally reported/recorded only to the *tenth* of a degree.

Exercises

Convert the following temperatures:

1. 35.4 °C = _________ °F

2. 103.6 °F = ________ °C

3. 96°F = ___________ °C

4. 44°C = ___________ °F

Math Assessment Test

I. Express in Roman numerals:

1. 14 ___________
2. 8 1/2 ___________
3. 36 ___________
4. 25 ___________

II. Express in Arabic numbers:

1. XIII ___________
2. XXIXss ___________
3. XLII ___________
4. XXXVIII ___________

III. Reduce the following factors to the lowest terms:

1. 15/25 ___________
2. 8/28 ___________
3. 12/52 ___________
4. 20/55 ___________

IV. Change the following improper fractions to whole or mixed numbers. Reduce to the lowest terms:

1. 11/2 ___________
2. 17/6 ___________
3. 17/7 ___________
4. 13/8 ___________

V. Change the following mixed numbers to improper fractions:

1. 3 5/9 ___________
2. 6 4/13 ___________
3. 5 3/16 ___________
4. 8 5/14 ___________

VI. Circle the larger fraction in each pair:

1. 6/13 or 9/13
2. 3/7 or 8/11
3. 8/11 or 8/19
4. 4/15 or 6/7

VII. Circle the smaller fraction in each pair:

1. 8/17 or 4/17
2. 2/11 or 2/13
3. 6/13 or 7/16

VIII. Add the following fractions and mixed numbers, and reduce to the lowest terms:

1. 4 2/5 + 2 1/2 + 3/4
2. 4 2/3 + 1/4 + 5/6
3. 9 2/3 + 3 2/5 + 3/4

IX. Subtract the following fractions:

1. 2 1/4 - 1 1/3
2. 5 1/2 - 1 1/3
3. 6 1/4 - 6 1/6

X. Multiply the following fractions and mixed numbers:

1. 3 5/6 x 4 1/8 = ___________
2. 2 1/6 x 5 ½ = ___________
3. 1 2/4 x 7 = ___________
4. 5 1/3 x 2 6/8 = ___________

Fraction word problems:

1. A clinic purchased an electronic vital signs equipment for $2,000 with a yearly maintenance cost of 1/5 of the purchase price. How much is the annual maintenance cost for this equipment?

2. A patient weighs 150 pounds (lb). If he is to receive 5 mg of medication per 50 pounds of body weight, how many mg of medication will be prescribed?

XI. Change the following decimals to fractions and reduce to the lowest terms:

1. 0.125 = ___________ 3. 0.635 = ___________

2. 0.45 = ___________ 4. 0.007 = ___________

XII. Circle the larger of the two decimals:

1. 0.3 or 0.06

2. 0.02 or 0.025

3. .12 or 0.078

XIII. Rewrite the following fractions as ratios, percentages, and decimals:

FRACTION	RATIO	PERCENTAGE	DECIMAL
1. 2/5	= ___________	= ___________	= ___________
2. 2/9	= ___________	= ___________	= ___________
3. 8/28	= ___________	= ___________	= ___________
4. 6/15	= ___________	= ___________	= ___________

XIV. Solve the following percentage problems:

1. 6% of 85 = ___________

2. 0.8% of 132 = ___________

3. 1.8% of 28 = ___________

4. 0.09% of 68 = ___________

Percentage word problems:

1. A Hydrocortisone Cream has 2 milligrams (mg) of hydrocortisone per 100 mg of the compound. What is the actual percentage of hydrocortisone in the compound?

2. An Intravenous solution of D5RL has 5 grams (g) of dextrose in each of 100 mL solution. What is the percentage of Ringer's lactate in the solution?

XV. Solve for "X" in the following proportions:

1. 2 : 7 :: 5 : X/2
2. 1/2 : X :: 2/3 : 12
3. X/15 = 7/20
4. 13X : 3 :: 1/3 : 1/26
5. 3/4 = 5X/1.5
6. 3 : 14 :: 3/4 : X/3
7. X/5 = 3/8
8. 4/22 = 6/ X/2
9. 5 : 13 :: X/2 : 17
10. 8 : 12 :: 5 : 3X

Unit conversion word problems:

1. How many teaspoons (tsp) are in 1 pint of medication preparation?

2. If there are 12 mg in a tablespoon (Tbs) of cough syrup, how many mg are in 5 fluid ounces?

3. A physician orders a teaspoon (tsp) of oral medication twice a day. How many days will ½ of a pint last?

4. If a man weighs 220 pounds (lb), what is his weight in kilograms (kg)?

5. If a patient is to take 10 grains (gr) of aspirin for his headache, how many milligrams (mg) is he to take?

XVI. 1. Problem: ¾ mL = How many m? ___________

2. Problem: gtt XV = How many m? ___________

3. Problem: 5/6 gr = How many mg? ___________

4. Problem: How many mL in 3 oz? ___________

5. Problem: 0.5 mg = How many mcg? ___________

6. Problem: 35 gtt = How many mL? ___________

7. Problem: How many cc in 3 qt? ___________

8. Problem: 4 gal = How many qt? ___________

9. Problem: 1.5 cup = How many cc? ___________

10. Problem: 24 oz = How many glasses? ___________

XVII. Convert the following to the equivalent measures indicated:

1. 0.002 kg = ___________ mg
2. 6.5 tbs = ___________ oz
3. 220 lbs = ___________ Kg
4. gr iiiss = ___________ mg
5. 0.480 L = ___________ pt
6. 3½ tbs = ___________ tsp
7. 35.4 °C = ___________ °F
8. 45 mL = ___________ dr
9. dr xxviiss = ___________ m
10. 103.6 °F = ___________ °C
11. 84 lbs = ___________ Kg
12. 120 cm = ___________ in
13. 0.135 L = ___________ mL
14. 60 gtts = ___________ tsp
15. 96°F = ___________ °C
16. 17.5 cm = ___________ in
17. 7 mL = ___________ gtts
18. 150 mg = ___________ g
19. 4 qt = ___________ mL
20. 3.05 g = ___________ mg
21. 0.45 g = ___________ gr
22. 44°C = ___________ °F
23. 65 Kg = ___________ lbs
24. 3.5 qt = ___________ L

Convert from traditional times to 24-Hr time or vice versa:

1. 10:45 pm = ____________ hrs.
2. 12:00 (midnight) = ____________ hrs.
3. 5:27 am = ____________ hrs.
4. 11:15 am = ____________ hrs.
5. 0215 hrs. = ____________
6. 2355 hrs. = ____________
7. 1020 hrs. = ____________
8. 1530 hrs. = ____________

Math Assessment Test - Answer Key

I. Express in Roman numerals:

1. 14 XIV
2. 8 1/2 VIIIss
3. 36 XXXVI
4. 25 XXV

II. Express in Arabic numbers:

1. XIII 13
2. XXIXss 29 1/2
3. XLII 42
4. XXXVIII 38

III. Reduce the following factors to the lowest terms:

1. 15/25 3/5
2. 8/28 2/7
3. 12/52 3/13
4. 20/55 4/11

IV. Change the following improper fractions to whole or mixed numbers. Reduce to the lowest terms:

1. 11/2 5 1/2
2. 17/6 2 5/6
3. 17/7 2 3/7
4. 13/8 1 5/8

V. Change the following mixed numbers to improper fractions:

1. 3 5/9 32/9
2. 6 4/13 82/13
3. 5 3/16 83/16
4. 8 5/14 117/14

VI. Circle the larger fraction in each pair:

1. 6/13 or (9/13)
2. 3/7 or (8/11)
3. (8/11) or 8/19
4. 4/15 or (6/7)

VII. Circle the smaller fraction in each pair:

1. 8/17 or (4/17)

2. 2/11 or (2/13)

3. 6/13 or (7/16)

VIII. Add the following fractions and mixed numbers, and reduce to the lowest terms:

1.
```
   4 2/5
   2 1/2
+    3/4
--------
 7 13/20
```

2.
```
   4 2/3
     1/4
+    5/6
--------
   5 3/4
```

3.
```
   9 2/3
   3 2/5
+    3/4
--------
13 49/60
```

IX. Subtract the following fractions:

1.
```
   2 1/4
-  1 1/3
--------
   11/12
```

2.
```
       5 1/2
-      1 1/3
------------
25/6 or 4 1/6
```

3.
```
       6 1/4
-      6 1/6
------------
2/24 or 1/12
```

X. Multiply the following fractions and mixed numbers:

1. 3 5/6 x 4 1/8 = 15 13/16

2. 2 1/6 x 5 ½ = 11 11/12

3. 1 2/4 x 7 = 10 1/2

4. 5 1/3 x 2 6/8 = 14 2/3

Fraction word problems:

1. A clinic purchased an electronic vital signs equipment for $2,000 with a yearly maintenance cost of 1/5 of the purchase price. How much is the annual maintenance cost for this equipment?

   = $400

2. A patient weighs 150 pounds (lb). If he is to receive 5 mg of medication per 50 pounds of body weight, how many mg of medication will be prescribed?

   = 15mg

XI. Change the following decimals to fractions and reduce to the lowest terms:

1. 0.125 = 1/8
2. 0.45 = 9/20
3. 0.635 = 127/200
4. 0.007 = 7/1000

XII. Circle the larger of the two decimals:

1. (0.3) or 0.06
2. 0.02 or (0.025)
3. (.12) or 0.078

XIII. Rewrite the following fractions as ratios, percentages, and decimals:

	FRACTION	RATIO	PERCENTAGE	DECIMAL
1.	2/5	= 2:5	= 40%	= 0.40
2.	2/9	= 2:9	= 22%	= 0.22
3.	8/28	= 8:28 or 2:7	= 29%	= 0.29
4.	6/15	= 6:15 or 2:5	= 40%	= 0.40

XIV. Solve the following percentage problems:

1. 6% of 85 = 5.1
2. 0.8% of 132 = 1.056
3. 1.8% of 28 = 0.504
4. 0.09% of 68 = 0.0612

Percentage word problems:

1. A Hydrocortisone Cream has 2 milligrams (mg) of hydrocortisone per 100 mg of the compound. What is the actual percentage of hydrocortisone in the compound?

   = 2%

2. An Intravenous solution of D5RL has 5 grams (g) of dextrose in each of 100 mL solution. What is the percentage of Ringer's lactate in the solution?

   = 5%

Solve for "X" in the following proportions:

1. 2 : 7 :: 5 : X/2 — X = 35
2. 1/2 : X :: 2/3 : 12 — X = 9
3. X/15 = 7/20 — X = 5.25
4. 13X : 3 :: 1/3 : 1/26 — X = 2
5. 3/4 = 5X/1.5 — X = 0.225
6. 3 : 14 :: 3/4 : X/3 — X = 10.5
7. X/5 = 3/8 — X = 1 7/8
8. 4/22 = 6/ X/2 — X = 66
9. 5 : 13 :: X/2 : 17 — X = 13 1/13
10. 8 : 12 :: 5 : 3X — X = 2.5

Unit conversion word problems:

1. How many teaspoons (tsp) are in 1 pint of medication preparation?

   = 96 tsp

2. If there are 12 mg in a tablespoon (Tbs) of cough syrup, how many mg are in 5 fluid ounces?

   = 120 mg

3. A physician orders a teaspoon (tsp) of oral medication twice a day. How many days will ½ of a pint last?

   = 21 ½ days

4. If a man weighs 220 pounds (lb), what is his weight in kilograms (kg)?

   = 100 pounds (lb)

5. If a patient is to take 10 grains (gr) of aspirin for his headache, how many milligrams (mg) is he to take?

   = 600 mg

XV.

1. Problem: ¾ mL = How many m? 11 1/4 m
2. Problem: gtt XV = How many m? 15 m
3. Problem: 5/6 gr = How many mg? 50 mg
4. Problem: How many mL in 3 oz? 90 mL
5. Problem: 0.5 mg = How many mcg? 500 mcg
6. Problem: 35 gtt = How many mL? 2 1/3
7. Problem: How many cc in 3 qt? 2880 cc
8. Problem: 4 gal = How many qt? 16 qt
9. Problem: 1.5 cup = How many cc? 180 cc
10. Problem: 24 oz = How many glasses? 4 glasses

XVI. Convert the following to the equivalent measures indicated:

1. 0.002 kg = 2000 mg
2. 6.5 tbs = 3.25 oz
3. 220 lbs = 100 Kg
4. gr iiiss = 210 mg
5. 0.480 L = 1 pt
6. 3½ tbs = 10.5 tsp
7. 35.4 °C = 95.7 °F

13. 0.135 L = 135 mL
14. 60 gtts = 0.8 tsp
15. 96°F = 35.6 °C
16. 17.5 cm = 6.9 in
17. 7 mL = 105 gtts
18. 150 mg = 0.150 g
19. 4 qt = 3840 mL

8. 45 mL = 9 dr

9. dr xxviiss = 2062.5 m

10. 103.6 °F = 39.8 °C

11. 84 lbs = 38.18 Kg

12. 120 cm = 47.2 in

20. 3.05 g = 3050 mg

21. 0.45 g = 7.5 gr

22. 44°C = 111.2 °F

23. 65 Kg = 143 lbs

24. 3.5 qt = 3.36 L

Convert from traditional times to 24-hr time or vice versa:

1. 10:45 pm = 2245 hrs.

2. 12:00 (midnight) = 2400 or 0000 hrs.

3. 5:27 am = 0527 hrs.

4. 11:15 am = 1115 hrs.

5. 0215 hrs. = 2:15 AM

6. 2355 hrs. = 11:55 PM

7. 1020 hrs. = 10:20 AM

8. 1530 hrs. = 3:30 PM

About the Author

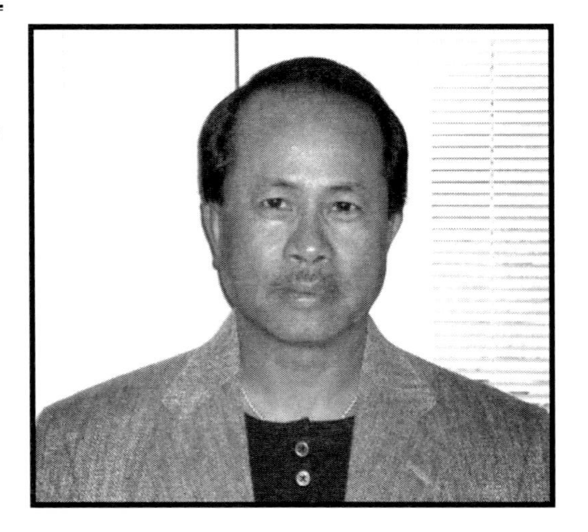

Louie Asuncion retired from the U.S. Navy in 1998 after twenty-four years of service as a Hospital Corpsman, Aviation Medicine Technician, Hospital Corpsman Instructor, and Independent Duty Corpsman (IDC). Having served in all types of navy ships and fighter squadrons and with the Marines, he is a veteran of the Vietnam era and Operation Desert Shield.

He has been teaching in Del Mar College's Nursing Education Department for ten years.

About TSTC Publishing

Established in 2004 as the publishing arm of the Texas State Technical College System, TSTC Publishing offers authors throughout the country the opportunity to initiate and participate in a variety of book development projects. Of course, in the twenty-first century, a book is no longer "just" a book, so TSTC Publishing projects now include such ancillary products as instructor guides, student workbooks, CD-ROMs, DVDs, ebooks and companion websites. In addition to offering editorial help and guidance to authors, assistance also is available in the areas of materials, production, distribution and sales.

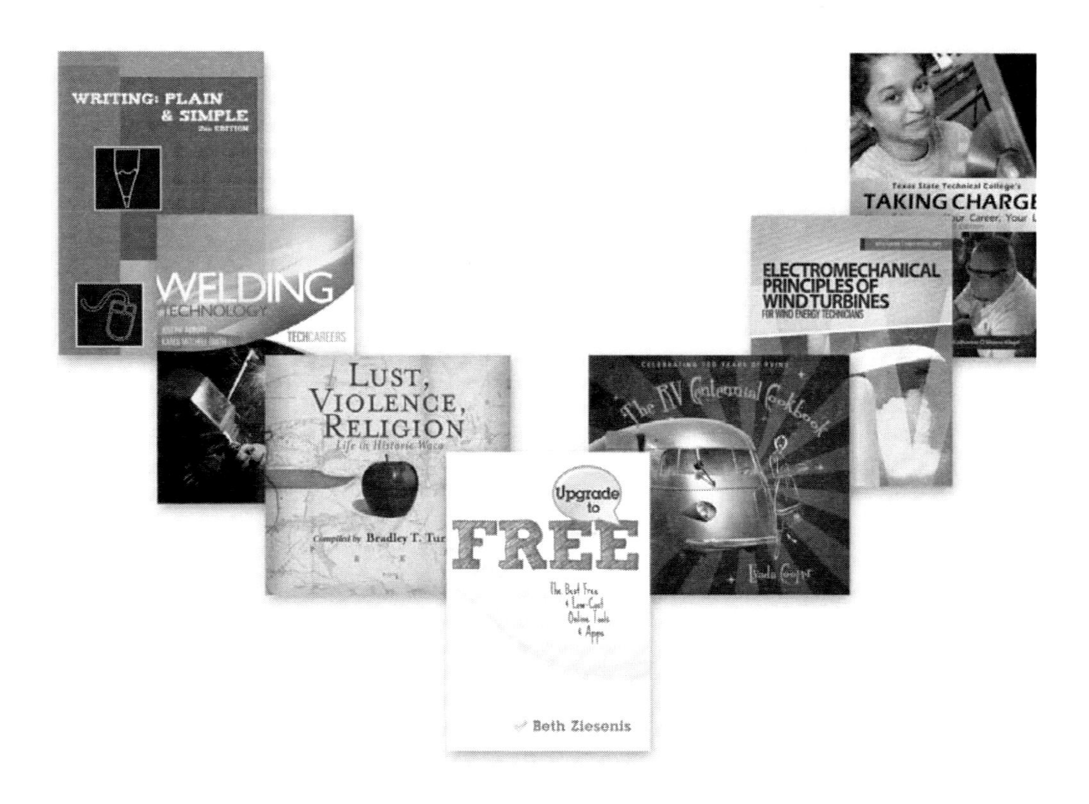